THE WOMEN BEFORE YOU

Wisdom To Navigate Your Fertility Challenge

Amy McKissick, NP-C

DEDICATION

To my seven sweet babies,

Anticipating the day I will gaze into your beautiful eyes and discover all your unique traits.

And I apologize if you inherited my curly hair.

ACKNOWLEDGEMENT

This book would not have been possible without the love and support of my beloved husband, Drew.

You are and will always be "my favorite".

TABLE OF CONTENTS

THE WOMAN WITH YOU

"Above all, be the heroine of your life, not the victim"
Nora Ephron

The ladies you will read about in this book about are my inspiration.

They have been where I am now.

They have been where I want to be.

They have overcome fertility challenges to give birth to healthy sons.

I am sure their lives were not easy. I am sure they had days where they cried, screamed, and wondered why they were not pregnant and having babies.

I know because I have done all of these things.

However, they declined to be a victim.

Just like these ladies, I decline to be a victim of fertility challenges.

I grew up thinking I would be "normal". After all, my mom had five children without any difficulties. There was no reason to think I would be any different.

I thought I would follow the pattern of many women before me—

Marriage
Career
Children

Initially, my life looked like it would not deviate from the pattern. I married at twenty-six and was attending graduate school for my Family Nurse Practitioner degree.

However, becoming pregnant remained elusive.

Although I wondered why I had not become pregnant, I never fully investigated it. I just reasoned that it would eventually happen. However, one night in December 2001 changed everything.

I had not been feeling well for a while—just some vague abdominal pain. Then one evening I woke up from sleep with excruciating right lower abdominal pain. My first thought—an appendicitis.

In the middle of this awful pain, I clearly heard God's voice telling me to seek medical care. I went to the emergency room where I had a CT scan which revealed a large cyst on my left ovary. The combination of the size of the mass and the leakage of blood was the root cause of the abdominal pain.

I left the emergency room with a prescription for pain medication, a follow-up appointment with my OB-GYN and a lot of questions swirling around in my mind. At the follow-up appointment, I had blood work and an ultrasound. He wanted to treat me with oral contraceptive pills and monitor the size of the ovarian cyst on surveillance ultrasounds over the next couple months. The thought behind this treatment was that the oral contraceptive pills would cause the cyst to shrink and disappear on its own.

However, when my blood work results came back this plan was thrown out the window.

One of the labs was a screening test for ovarian cancer. He did not believe it would be elevated, but had drawn it just as a precaution. This test came back significantly elevated. Due to this result, he now advised surgery…within the next twenty-four hours.

As I sat in his office later that day signing the consent for surgery, I was agreeing to give him carte blanche.

Because it was unclear what was causing the abnormal result, I had to consent to give him permission to do whatever was necessary. Even if that meant removing all my reproductive organs. That was a sobering moment.

What if I awoke to find out I could not have children?

How would this affect my marriage?

How would I recover from the trauma of mourning children I would never have?

However, there was such a tangible presence of the Holy Spirit during all of this.

During surgery the next day, the decision was made to send a portion of the cyst to pathology while I was still on the operating table. Thank God, the pathology report was benign.

The surgery revealed the cyst was actually an endometrioma, which is a large blood-filled cyst, caused by endometriosis. The endometriosis had also caused significant inflammation in my abdomen. This was the reason the blood test for ovarian cancer came back abnormal. It was detecting the inflammation from the endometriosis.

The surgery was a complete success at removing the endometrioma and the adhesions from the endometriosis. However, since endometriosis thrives on estrogen to grow, the decision was made to start treatment with Depo-Lupron injections. I would get the first injection upon discharge from the hospital.

Let me tell you—Depo Lupron injections are not for the faint of heart!

It shuts down all the estrogen production in your body in less than twenty-four hours. This means you don't ease into menopause. You get there in warp speed!

I distinctly remember being curled up in the fetal position on my sofa because of the headache that resulted from all the estrogen being sucked out of my body.

Over the next twenty years it has been a blur of fertility treatments, miscarriages and conversations with God. Through all of it, He has reassured me that I can trust Him, His Word is still true, and that a diagnosis does not define who I am. He also has reminded me that I am not the first woman to face fertility challenges.

Maybe you just discovered you might have a challenge with fertility.

Maybe you have been dealing with fertility challenges for years.

I have been where you are.

It is my sincere hope that this book provides answers to your questions, encouragement for your soul and hope in the middle of your fertility challenge.

I am the woman with you.

CAN I TRUST YOU?

"Never be afraid to trust an unknown future to a known God"

Corrie ten Boom

This is a question I always ask myself when I am introduced to a new person. And the initial answer is always the same.

"Not Yet".

Trust is a sacred commodity. It is in short supply and not easy to source. No one should be granted that level of access into your life without first going through a lengthy vetting process. Failure to do so can result in catastrophic damage. This I know from personal experience.

I have made the mistake of granting trust to friends, colleagues, and men way too early. By doing so, it led to months of physical, emotional, and financial recovery. If I had only waited longer and carefully observed their flawed character and how their words did not match up with their actions, I could have avoided a lot of damage.

Experiences like these can tempt you into becoming skeptical and bitter. Maybe you are at a point where you don't want to trust anyone—including God. After all, people that you can see and interact with have failed you in the past. So, you may be wondering, "How can I trust a God that I can't physically see to heal my body and give me a child?".

This is a valid question.

In fact, God doesn't mind you asking the question and He is happy to answer it.

Questions indicate you are willing to learn more and give God a chance to explain some things to you. The only way to develop trust with anyone, including God, is to spend time with them.

Evaluate their character.

Listen to their words.

Observe their actions.

As you do these things over a period of time, you will be able to determine whether or not they treat people fairly, honor their words, and follow through on their commitments. Then you can make an informed decision regarding granting them your trust.

So, if you apply the above criteria to God, would you make the decision to trust Him? I believe the answer is a resounding, "Yes!".

The Bible has numerous verses that speak about God's character, words, and actions that provide evidence that He can be trusted.

His Character

Everybody has character, including God.

A person's character provides insight to how he will behave in a given situation. Unfortunately, some will change their behavior based on who may, or may not, be watching at that particular moment. God is not one of those people. His character is consistent and unchanging. This is evidenced by the below Scriptures—

"For I am The Lord, I change not…"

Malachi 3:6 (KJV)

"God is not human, that He should lie, not being a human being, that He should change His mind. Does He speak and then not act? Does He promise and not fulfill?"

Numbers 23:19 (NIV)

"Every good and perfect gift is from above, coming down from The Father of the heavenly lights, who does not change like shifting shadows."

James 1:17 (NIV)

His Word

In today's society, it seems that most people don't think twice about not following through on the word they have promised to someone. Thankfully, God is not like this. He has revealed to us the importance He places on His Word.

"The Lord said to me, "You have seen correctly, for I am watching to see that My Word is fulfilled."

Jeremiah 1:12 (NIV)

"It is the same with My Word. I send it out and it always produces fruit. It will accomplish all I want it to, and it will prosper everywhere I send it."

Isaiah 55:11 (NLT)

"I will worship toward Your holy temple, And praise Your Name for Your Lovingkindness and Your Truth; For You have magnified Your Word above Your Name."

Psalm 138:2 (NKJV)

"For I truly tell you, until Heaven and Earth disappear, not the smallest letter, not the least stroke of a pen, will by any means disappear from the Law until everything is accomplished."

Matthew 5:18 (NIV)

His Action

One of the primary ways God acts is through His spoken Word. This is how He created the world and mankind. The words God speaks are a clear indicator of what is in His heart. (Matt 12:34; Luke 6:45) It reveals the true value He places on people and situations they are facing. God has provided us with evidence of His Word to address fertility.

"So God created man in His own image, in the image and likeness of God He created him; male and female He created them. And God blessed them and said to them, Be fruitful, multiply, and fill the earth, and subdue it (using all its vast resources in the service of God and man); and have dominion over the fish of the sea, the birds of the air, and over every living creature that moves upon the earth.'

Genesis 1:27-28 (AMP)

"And you, be fruitful and multiply, bring forth abundantly on the earth and multiply on it"

Genesis 9:7 (AMP)

"None shall lose her young by miscarriage or be barren in your land; I will fulfill the number of your days"

Exodus 23:26 (AMP)

"You shall be blessed above all peoples; there shall not be male or female barren among you or among your cattle"

Deuteronomy 17:14 (AMP)

"Then Elisha went to the spring of the waters and cast the salt in it and said, Thus says The Lord: I (not the salt) have healed these waters; there shall not be any more death, miscarriage, or barreness (and bereavement) because of it. So the waters were healed to this day, as Elisha had said"

2 Kings 2:21-22 (AMP)

These Scriptures provide substantial evidence that God not only meets, but exceeds, the requirements to be granted your trust. However, He won't make you trust Him. It has to be a decision you make of your own free will. But once you do, you will begin to see Him do amazing things in your life.

IT'S NOT YOUR FAULT

"The truth will set you free, but first it will piss you off"
Joe Klauss

Most of my life I had this nagging feeling that everything that went wrong in my life was my fault. I realize this sounds ridiculous. However, being rational rarely enters into the discussion when I am over analyzing a situation!

So naturally, when I started having difficulty conceiving and experiencing miscarriages there had to be only one answer—

"It was my fault".

The running conversation in my head went something like this—

"If I wasn't so stressed from work, I would be pregnant by now."

"If I hadn't tripped and fell, I would not have miscarried."

"If I took all those vitamins, I would be pregnant again by now."

And then there is the one thought that tortures me and every other Christian woman—

"If I had more faith, none of this would be happening to me."

These are just some of the conversations I have had with myself. Yours may sound similar or completely different.

Maybe you think the abortion you had in college, the affair you had with a married man, or the decision to delay having children so you could focus on your career are the reasons you are having challenges with fertility.

Regardless of the thoughts running through your mind, they all originate from the one core belief— "It's my fault".

But what if it's not?

What if there is someone actively working against you?

Someone who doesn't want you to become pregnant and have healthy children?

I know it sounds unbelievable to think such a horrible individual exists. Seriously, who would be that evil and callous?

The truth is that someone is doing exactly that. And that someone is the devil. It really should not be a surprise to discover he is behind all of this. After all, this has been his mode of operation for centuries.

Jesus told us this Himself. He told us that the devil's mission is to accomplish three things in our lives—steal, kill and destroy.

So, when your fertility is being attacked and your children are dying through a miscarriage, then you know this is his work.

"The thief comes only to steal and kill and destroy. I have come that they may have life and have it to the full"

John 10:10 (NIV)

The devil's plan to interfere with a woman's fertility didn't start with you. It actually started back in Genesis with Eve. After Adam and Eve disobeyed God, listened to the lie of the devil, and ate from the tree of the knowledge of good and evil, then God's judgement came.

To the serpent (the devil)—

"And The Lord God said to the serpent, Because you have done this, you are cursed above all (domestic) animals and above every (wild) living thing of the field; upon your belly you shall go, and you shall eat dust (and what it contains) all the days of your life. And I will put enmity between you and the woman, and between your offspring and her Offspring; He will bruise and tread your head underfoot, and you will lie in wait and bruise His heel"

Genesis 3:14-15 (AMP)

Notice that God said there would be "enmity" between the devil and Eve. Enmity is a strong word. It means a lot more than they won't "like" each other. Enmity is defined as—

"the state or feeling of being actively opposed or hostile to someone or something".

The enmity wasn't self-limiting to Eve and the devil. It would continue for all generations to come. So, you can see that the devil is actively opposing you in every area of your life—including your fertility.

To Eve—

"To the woman He said, I will greatly multiply your grief and your suffering in pregnancy and the pangs of childbearing; with spasms of distress you will bring forth children. Yet your desire and craving will be for your husband, and he will rule over you."

Genesis 3:16 (AMP)

So, God told Eve she would have challenges during pregnancy and childbirth. There would be pain involved.

However, He NEVER SAID she would be barren or experience a miscarriage!

It's Not All About You

It may feel like your fertility challenges only involve you and your husband. But there are bigger stakes involved than just the two of you. Spiritual things are never just about the two people involved at a moment in time. It always involves the impact it will have on the generations to come.

The Bible does not tell us that Eve had a problem conceiving Cain and Able. But just a few generations later in Genesis 16, we can see the curse at work. It is the first time we see a woman facing fertility challenges. And that woman is Sarai.

So why Sarai?

Because she is the wife of Abram. He will become Abraham and the father to the nation of Israel. She will become Sarah and give birth to Isaac who is in the ancestral line of Jesus Christ. If the devil can stop the birth of Isaac in Genesis 21, then he thinks he can stop the birth of Jesus later in Matthew 1, Mark 2 and Luke 2.

So why you?

Because your child has a destiny on their life. The devil wants to stop him or her from being born so their destiny is never fulfilled. The best way to stop someone from fulfilling their destiny is to make sure they are never born.

So, he interferes with your fertility.

You Can Play Offense

At this point, you might think that you have no weapons to fight back against the devil. Nothing could be further from the truth. Just because the devil tries to prevent you from conceiving and bearing healthy children, doesn't mean he has to succeed. You have two very effective weapons at your disposal.

In fact, they are the same weapons that Jesus Himself used against the devil—

The Word and delegated authority.

The Word

Remember in Chapter One when God told us He honors His Word above His own Name? (Psalm 138:2 (NKJV).

Jesus remembered it.

In fact, it is what He used to defeat the devil during His temptation in the wilderness. He told the devil, "It is written", "It is written", and "It is said" three times in Luke. (Luke 4:4, 8, 12 KJV) Jesus knows The Word and He knows the power it contains to silence the devil. When Jesus spoke The Word, it was the same as if God Himself had spoken it.

It is the same for us today.

When we speak The Word in faith, it is the same as God Himself is speaking it.

"For the Word of God is quick, and powerful, and sharper than any two-edged sword, piercing even to the dividing asunder of soul and spirit, and of the joints and marrow, and is a discerner of the thoughts and intents of the heart"

Hebrews 4:12 (KJV)

You will have to use The Word repeatedly to attack the devil. Jesus had to do this and He is The Son of God. Since Jesus had to use The Word more than once against the devil, don't be discouraged when you have to do the same.

The reason you will have to consistently use The Word against the devil is because he is determining whether or not you know who you are as a Christian and whether you believe The Scripture for yourself.

His temptation of Jesus failed.

Sometimes his temptation of us succeeds.

However, his success does not mean The Word does not work. It only means we need to become as convinced as Jesus is regarding the power in The Word.

Delegated Authority

Now that you understand the power of The Word, it is imperative that you understand that you have the delegated authority to use it in Jesus' name. Jesus had delegated authority from God to do things on His behalf while He was on the earth. Likewise, as a Christian, you can use Jesus' name and all His resources to resolve any issue that arises in your life.

Jesus delegated His authority to His disciples numerous times when He was on the earth.

Below is one example.

"After these things The Lord appointed other seventy also, and sent them two and two before His face into every city and place, whither He Himself would come. And the seventy returned again with joy, saying, "Lord, even the devils are subject unto us through Thy Name. And He said unto them, I beheld Satan as lightning fall from heaven. Behold, I give unto you power to tread on serpents and scorpions, and over all the power of the enemy: and nothing shall by any means hurt you. Notwithstanding in this rejoice not, that the spirits are subject unto you; but rather rejoice because your names are written in heaven."

Luke 10:1, 17-20 (KJV)

The greatest example of delegated authority is The Great Commission. This is where Jesus gave The Church their mission on the earth after He ascended to Heaven.

"Go then and make disciples of all the nations, baptizing them into the name of The Father and of The Son and of The Holy Spirit, teaching them to observe everything that I have commanded you, and behold, I am with you all the days (perpetually, uniformly, and on every occasion, to the (very) close and consummation of the age. Amen (so be it)."

Matthew 28:19-20 (AMP)

"And He said to them, Go into all the world and preach and publish openly the good news (The Gospel) to every creature (of the whole human race). He who believes (who adheres to and trusts in and relies on The Gospel and Him Whom it sets forth) and is baptized will be saved (from the penalty of eternal death); but he who does not believe (who does not adhere to and trust in and rely on The Gospel and Him Whom is sets forth) will be condemned. And these attesting signs will accompany those who believe: in My name they will drive out demons, they will speak in new languages; they will pick up serpents; and (even) if they drink anything deadly, it will not hurt them; they will lay their hands on the sick, and they will get well."

Mark 16:15-18 (AMP)

If delegated authority seems like a foreign concept, just think about an ambassador. An ambassador represents his country to a foreign nation. He has powers that are given, or delegated, to him by the President of his country. He uses this delegated authority and the name of the President to ensure the President's will is accomplished when interacting with a foreign nation.

As a Christian, you are an ambassador for Jesus Christ (2 Cor 5:20).

You have the delegated authority to use The Word the same way Jesus did. Because you have a covenant relationship with Jesus you can find scripture regarding your fertility, submit yourself to God, use The Word against the devil, and he has to stop attacking you (James 4:7).

It is important to realize that the devil no longer has control in the earth over Christians.

He had power over all the earth after Adam and Eve sinned. However, his power was stripped away from him when Jesus was resurrected from the dead. So, now the only way the devil can have power in our lives is by taking advantage of our ignorance that Jesus has already defeated him on our behalf. He uses our ignorance against us to gain access to our lives.

"Jesus approached and, breaking the silence, said to them, All authority (all power of rule) in heaven and on earth has been given to Me."

Matthew 28:18 (AMP)

"Beware lest any man spoil you through philosophy and vain deceit, after the tradition of men, after the rudiments of the world, and not after Christ. For in Him dwelleth all the fullness of The Godhead bodily. And ye are complete in Him, which is the head of all principality and power."

Colossians 2:8-10 (KJV)

"When He (God) had disarmed the rulers and authorities [those supernatural forces of evil operating against us], He made a public example of them [exhibiting them as captives in His triumphal procession], having triumphed over them through the cross."

Colossians 2:15 (AMP)

"And The Ever-living One (I am living in the eternity of the eternities). I died, but see, I am alive forevermore; and I possess the keys of death and Hades (the realm of the dead).

Revelation 1:18 (AMP)

Now you know the real enemy of your fertility.

Now you know the weapons you have available to use against him.

So, what are you going to do with this information?

Knowledge without action will never change your situation. The next time the devil tries to torment you about your fertility, open your mouth, and respond to him by speaking Scripture.

This will shut him up every time!

YOU ARE NOT A DIAGNOSIS

"Define yourself radically as one beloved by God. This is the true self. Every other identity is illusion."

Brennan Manning

"Tell me about yourself".

When you meet someone for the first time, they will inevitably ask about your life and your profession. I personally hate this question. Attempting to sum up my life into an elevator pitch is ridiculous.

So, where would I start?

"Married at 26. NP degree at 31. Widow at 39. Remarried at 42. Fertility challenges x 20 years."

If your default answer includes information about your fertility challenges, then you have subconsciously started identifying with a diagnosis.

You probably don't even realize you are doing it. It is an easy default, because fertility treatment consumes a large portion of your time, finances and emotional reserves. Eliminating the discussion of fertility topics from my casual social conversations has been something I have actively pursued in my own life over the last few years.

It is not that you don't talk about fertility issues with other people. You do need a close group of people that can walk with you through this challenge. But those people are not random individuals at a social event.

You may have noticed that I don't use the term "infertility".

This is a conscious, calculated decision on my part.

I have discovered during my decades of clinical practice that when people heavily focus on a diagnosis it becomes part of their identity. Their vision becomes obscured and all they can see is the diagnosis. They forget all the other wonderful parts of their life and the characteristics that make them unique.

A diagnosis does not define you—unless you allow it to.

So how can you tell if you have crossed the line?

There are a few red flags that should warn you that your focus on fertility has become too microscopic—

#1-Social conversations with acquaintances involve a discussion of fertility .

#2-Planning leisure activities and travel involve a discussion on whether it would harm a baby (just in case you are pregnant and don't know it yet).

#3-Decisions on career based on insurance coverage for fertility treatments.

#4-Decision to have sex with your husband is based on an ovulation test.

When you see these things start to occur, you can know that a diagnosis is attempting to become your identity. It's time to take a step back and evaluate your true identity.

Who Are You?

If your identity is not a diagnosis, what is it based on?

Your marriage?

Your career?

Your social circle?

All of these things are subject to change.

A death could end your marriage.

A layoff could derail your career.

A move could change your social circle.

Then who are you?

If your identity is not based on what you can see with your eyes, then what is it based on? Your identity has to be based on something that is eternally secure. It has to be based on who God said you are in Scripture.

First, He told us who we are—

"So God created man in His own image, in the image and likeness of God He created Him; male and female He created them"

Genesis 1:27 (AMP)

Then, He told us what we have—

"Namely, the righteousness of God which comes by believing with personal trust and confident reliance on Jesus Christ (the Messiah). [And it is meant] for all who believe. For there is no distinction"

Romans 3:22 (AMP)

Therefore, you know that your identity is made up of two immutable things: being made in the image and likeness of God and that you are the righteousness of God through your relationship with Jesus Christ. A diagnosis will come and go, but your identity remains steadfast.

THE WOMEN BEFORE YOU

"There are years that ask questions and years that answer."

Zora Neale Hurston

When you are in the middle of dealing with fertility issues, it feels like a struggle that will never end. Each month holds the hope of a positive pregnancy test which is all too often followed by the disappointment of another menstrual cycle. It results in a monthly grieving process that only those who have faced the same challenge can truly understand.

Thankfully, there are women who have walked this path before you. Each willing to impart their wisdom to you. To bare their souls and share their entire story with you—including the parts that demonstrate their doubt and desperation. All in an effort to help you with your fertility challenge.

SARAH

"AMA"

This dreaded acronym means "Advanced Maternal Age" and is the label the medical community uses to tag women who are either pregnant or deliver their baby at or after the age of 35 years. It means you are doing something that only women younger than you should be doing. In fact, you are engaging in a high-risk behavior as far as they are concerned.

They would have slapped this term on Sarah's medical chart in a hot second!

After all, she was 90 years old at the time she gave birth to Isaac. But Sarah probably didn't care what label someone put on her or what people were saying about her behind her back. She was finally pregnant!

God had promised Abram that he would have a child of his own. But decades later, Sarai still had not conceived. The shame associated with being unable to provide a child for her husband was acute.

The overwhelming desire for a child can make a woman do some crazy things. And Sarai was no different. Her crazy idea was this: "I will tell my husband to sleep with my maid, she will get pregnant, and the child will be his heir".

Unfortunately for all involved, sometimes crazy works.

So, when Abram is 86 years old Hagar gives birth to a son, Ishmael. But he was not the heir God had promised Abram.

Four years later, when Abram was 90 years old, God appeared to Abram and changed his name to Abraham. Abraham means "Father of many nations". He also told Abraham that He was changing Sarai's name to Sarah which means "Mother of nations" and that she would have a son.

God also went ahead and saved Abraham and Sarah the heated debate regarding picking out a name for their son. He told Abraham he was to name their son “Isaac” and he would be the child with whom He would establish His everlasting covenant to include all his descendants.

Ten years later, when Abraham was 100 years old, God’s promise was fulfilled. (Genesis 15-17, 21)

Wisdom from Sarah—
God always keeps His Word.

Trying to help God will complicate the situation.

Sometimes God will tell the husband, not the wife, about the upcoming pregnancy.

There can be decades between the promise and the birth.

Start calling yourself fertile before you become pregnant.

God knew the name of the child before he was formed.

God will tell you when the child is coming.

REBEKAH

Sarah's daughter-in-law would also face fertility challenges.

It was twenty years from the time Isaac prayed to The Lord regarding Rebekah being barren until the time she gave birth to twins, Esau and Jacob.

It is unclear how old Rebekah was at the time of her marriage. But we do know that Isaac was forty years old when he married Rebekah and he was sixty years old at the time the twins were born. (Genesis 24-25)

During the pregnancy, Rebekah experienced complications. The twins were struggling within her. This was concerning to her, so she asked The Lord about it.

"If it is so [that The Lord has heard our prayer], why am I like this? And she went to inquire of The Lord, and the Lord said unto her, [The founders of] two nations are in your womb, and the separation of two peoples has begun in your body; the one people shall be stronger than the other, and the elder shall serve the younger." Genesis 25:22-23 (AMP)

Wisdom from Rebekah—
God always keeps His Word.

A husband can intercede for his wife's fertility.

There can be decades between the promise and the birth.

Believe that God hears you when you pray. Sometimes He doesn't respond to you at that moment. Sometimes His response is the manifestation of what you prayed for.

Sometimes a pregnancy you have believed God for can have complications. Ask God and he will tell you want is happening with the pregnancy.

RACHEL

Rebekah's daughter-in-law would also face fertility challenges.

The Scriptures are silent regarding Rachel's age at the time of her marriage to Jacob or when Joseph was born. However, Scripture does tell us that she was barren for a period of time.

Rachel had an unusual marriage. In fact, she was involved in a polygamist relationship. Both she and her older sister, Leah, were married to Jacob. As you can imagine this caused a significant amount of rivalry between the sisters! This only intensified when Leah had multiple children and Rachel was yet to produce an heir.

Frustrated by the situation, Rachel confronts Jacob and tells him, "Give me children, or else I die" (Genesis 30:1 KJV). This is a perfect example of the level of frustration and desperation fertility issues can drive a woman!

Jacob responds by telling her He is not God and it's not his fault she is barren.

So, Rachel decides she will do what Sarah did—she wants her husband to sleep with her maid, Bilhah, so she can have children through her. Jacob didn't learn from the mistake of his grandfather, so he sleeps with the maid. Bilhah did conceive and produce two children with Jacob.

However, this did not satisfy Rachel's longing for a child of her own.

This caused her to engage in even more drastic measures to conceive. She negotiated with Leah and made her the following offer: A night with Jacob in exchange for the mandrakes Leah's son had harvested.

Why would Rachel offer Jacob to her sister in exchange for mandrakes? Because mandrakes were reported to have medicinal properties that aided in fertility. However, they were also poisonous.

After a period of time, "God remembered Rachel and answered her pleading and made it possible for her to have children. And [now for the first time] she became pregnant and bore a son; and she said, God has taken away my reproach, disgrace and humiliation. And she called his name Joseph [may he add] and said, May the Lord add to me another son". (Genesis 30:22-24 AMP)

It is interesting that God used the plural term, "children" when this was Rachel's first pregnancy. God knows the end from the beginning and He knew she would have more than one child.

And Rachel did have another son, Benjamin. However, she died during his birth. (Genesis 29-35)

Wisdom from Rachel—

God always keeps His Word.

Trying to help God give you a child will complicate the situation.

Don't repeat the same mistake your ancestor made.

Only God can open a womb and give a woman a child.

Don't put pressure on your husband to give you what only God can.

Resorting to alternative medicines to improve fertility can be dangerous.

MANOAH'S WIFE

The scriptures are silent regarding Manoah's wife's age at the time of Samson's birth. However, the scriptures do confirm that she was barren. The Angel of The Lord initially appears to her alone and gives her the following prophecy—

"And The Angel of The Lord appeared to the woman and said to her, Behold, you are barren and have no children, but you shall become pregnant and bear a son. Therefore, beware and drink no wine or strong drink and eat nothing unclean. For behold, you shall become pregnant and bear a son. No razor shall come upon his head, for the child shall be a Nazarite to God from birth and he shall begin to deliver Israel out of the hands of the Philistines."

Judges 13:3-5 (AMP)

I love the fact that The Angel of The Lord did not sugar coat the situation. He laid out the facts as they currently were. What I love more, is the fact that he told her the situation would change.

She tells her husband, Manoah, about the encounter and he asks God to send The Angel of The Lord back a second time to tell them how they are to raise the child. God grants his request. The second time The Angel of The Lord appears to the woman and this time she runs to get Manoah so he can hear the prophecy for himself.

This time The Angel of The Lord only repeats a portion of the prophecy—He does not repeat the part related to no razor coming upon his head, his Nazarite heritage or that he will begin to deliver Israel out of the hands of the Philistines. He simply says to them both "All that I commanded her let her observe" (Judges 13:14 AMP).

It is unclear the length of time from the above prophecy to the birth to Samson.

Wisdom from Manoah's wife—
God always keeps His Word.

God may tell you to avoid certain foods and drinks in preparation for pregnancy.

God won't repeat parts of a child's destiny to anyone else…even to his father.

HANNAH

The Scriptures are silent regarding the number of years Hannah was barren. However, oral Jewish tradition states it is believed she was barren for nineteen years. Hannah found herself in the same unenviable position as Rachel—in a polygamist relationship. Elkanah's other wife, Peninnah, had children. And she made sure to torture Hannah with this truth.

Elkanah found himself in the same position that Jacob did—the wife he loved was unable to have children.

Hannah was so upset by being unable to have children that she wept and would not eat. She was so troubled in her soul that she went to temple of The Lord to pray. This is the prayer she uttered:

"She vowed, saying, "O Lord of Hosts, if You will indeed look on the affliction of Your handmaid and [earnestly] remember, and not forget Your handmaid but will give me a son, I will give him to The Lord all his life; no razor shall touch his head".

1 Samuel 1:11 (AMP)

Eli, the high priest, saw Hannah praying and thought she was drunk because she was only moving her lips. However, the prayer was being uttered from her heart. Hannah explained the situation and he answered, "Then Eli said, Go in peace, and may the God of Israel grant your petition which you have asked of Him" (1 Samuel 1:17 AMP). Hannah believed she received the answer to her prayer as evidenced by her change in behavior. She resumed eating and was no longer sad.

Hannah did conceive and give birth to a son. She named him Samuel and kept him until he was weaned. Then she took him to Eli and dedicated him to The Lord. Samuel grew to become a prophet of The Lord and none of his words fell to the ground (1 Samuel 3:19-20). God continued to bless Hannah with an additional three sons and two daughters (1 Samuel 2:21).

Wisdom from Hannah—
God always keeps His Word.

A husband can't replace the longing in a woman's heart for children.

The desire for children can become unbalanced and result in emotional and physical distress.

Believing that your prayer has been granted when you pray will immediately change your behavior and countenance.

THE SHUNAMMITE WOMAN

The Scripture is silent about the age of The Shunammite Woman when she gives birth. It does tell us that she was rich, influential, and a supporter of the ministry of Elisha. She extended gracious hospitality to Elisha by having an addition built on her home so he could stay there and rest during his travels.

In an effort to repay her for her generosity, he offered to mention her to the king or to the commander of the army.

She declined.

But he was determined to bless her so he called his servant Gehazi to find out what might be a blessing to her. Gehazi replied, "She has no child and her husband is old" (2 Kings 4:14 AMP).

So, Elisha calls her back again and speaks the following prophecy over her—

"At this season when the time comes round, you shall embrace a son. She said, No, my lord, you man of God, do not lie to your handmaid."

2 Kings 4:16 (AMP)

She did not rejoice at this news. She had come to the point in her life where she stopped hoping for a child and just had accepted her life. But this did not stop Elisha's prophecy from being fulfilled.

"But the woman conceived and bore a son at that season the following year, as Elisha had said to her"

2 Kings 4:17 (AMP)

Wisdom from The Shunammite Woman—
God always keeps His Word.

Hospitality can put you in a position to receive the desire of your heart.

Years of fertility challenges can interfere with receiving from God.

ELISABETH

The Scriptures are silent regarding Elisabeth's age at the time of John the Baptist's birth, but it does say she and her husband, Zachariah were "both righteous" and "far advanced in years" (Luke 1: 6-7 AMP). Oral tradition states she was about sixty years when the birth occurred.

Zachariah was a priest and one day and while he was burning incense in The Temple of The Lord, the angel Gabriel appeared to him and gave him the following prophecy—

"But the angel said unto him, Fear not, Zacharias: for thy prayer is heard; and thy wife Elisabeth shall bear thee a son, and thou shalt call his name John. And thou shalt have joy and gladness; and many shall rejoice at his birth. For he shall be great in the sight of The Lord, and shall drink neither wine nor strong drink; and he shall be filled with The Holy Ghost, even from his mother's womb. And many of the children of Israel shall he turn to The Lord their God. And he shall go before Him in the spirit and power of Elias, to turn the hearts of the fathers to the children, and the disobedient to the wisdom of the just; to make ready a people prepared for The Lord".

Luke 1:13-17 (KJV)

Now as you can imagine, Zachariah was probably awestruck by a visitation from Gabriel and the prophecy he had just received. So, he asks for confirmation, "How can I be sure of this? I am an old man and my wife is well along in years." (Luke 1:18 NIV).

This question sounds very similar to the one Mary asked Gabriel about when he told her she would conceive Jesus. In Mary's case, the question was a valid question since she was a virgin. However, the question Zachariah asked was based in unbelief. So, Gabriel struck him dumb until the birth of John the Baptist.

After his assignment at The Temple was completed, Zachariah returned home to Elisabeth and she conceived. She remained secluded for the first five months of her pregnancy. Zachariah must have written a note to Elisabeth during her pregnancy explaining all that Gabriel had told him about their son.

When it was time for John the Baptist to be named, all those present called him "Zachariah" after his father. But Elisabeth corrected them and said the baby's name is "John". They didn't believe her so they asked Zachariah. He took a piece of paper and wrote the name "John" to confirm his name. Once he did this, he was able to speak again.

Wisdom from Elisabeth—
God always keeps His Word.

Righteous people can have fertility challenges.

Keep your mouth shut so you don't speak unbelief and interfere with his plan for your children.

Seclusion may be necessary to protect you and your pregnancy.

Your child's destiny may be tied to someone else's. Therefore, their birth may have to occur as a specific time to fulfill their destiny.

All these women lead remarkable lives and gave birth to some of the most important men in the history of Christianity. You may have noticed that each of the women's first borne children were males. Scripture tells us there is a special consecration on the first male that opens the womb.

"Sanctify (consecrate, set apart) to Me all the firstborn (males); whatever is first to open the womb among the Israelites, both of man and of beast, is Mine."

Exodus 13:2 (AMP)

It was a challenge for each of these women to conceive their sons. However, each of these men arrived on the earth at the precise time to fulfill their destiny. I am sure all these ladies would have preferred to have their children earlier in life. But what if they had? How would that have altered the course of history? We may not always understand the delay in the arrival of our children, but we can trust that God's timing is perfect.

RESOURCES

"Hannah's Miracle Child"

Many people know Marty as a personal trainer, nutrition specialist and fitness instructor. You may have heard her testimony of how God delivered her from overeating and eating disorders. What you may not know is that Marty struggled both to get pregnant and to maintain healthy pregnancies.

When Marty Copeland studied the story of Hannah, she had an instant realization. Hannah had great faith and believed God would give her a son, and He did. Marty knew God is no respecter of persons. If He opened Hannah's womb and she conceived, Marty realized He could do the same for her. That's all she needed to get on the road to believing God for her own children.

Whatever you're believing God for, whether it's a happy marriage, a godly husband or an increase in your finances, don't give up. Set your faith to have the same stance as Hannah, and don't let go until you get what is rightfully yours! (courtesy http://www.kcm.org)

This product is available from www.kcm.org

"No More Sad"

Pastor Keith Moore examines the story of Hannah from an entirely new perspective. After listening to this teaching, you will view the diagnosis of infertility differently and be "no more sad."

This teaching is available free at www.moorelife.org

"Redeemed From the Curse of Sickness"

Sickness in any part of your body is a curse. It can manifest as a common cold, a reproductive disorder, or a terminal illness. Regardless of how it shows up in your life, you don't have to receive it. Jesus redeemed you from the curse of sickness through his death, burial and resurrection. In this in-depth study, Pastor Keith Moore explains exactly what the curse of sickness is and how you don't have to experience sickness in any part of your body.

This series is available free at www.moorelife.org

"Vision of Victory"

If you can see it, you can do it; if you can see it, you can be it; if you can see it, you can have it. Your vision is like a blueprint inside you. You have to see it on the inside of you before it will ever happen on the outside. Pastor Keith Moore tells you how to get the right vision inside of you in this four-message series. Learn the dynamics of natural seeing and spiritual seeing, how your faith will produce your vision, and how what you behold is what you become. Get a vision for your victory so your faith can get to work on it today. (Courtesy moorelife.org) This series is available free at www.moorelife.org

SCRIPTURES

Have you ever wondered what God has to say on the subject of fertility? Below you will read directly from His Word what He has to say about it…and trust me, He has plenty to say on the subject!

I encourage you to meditate on and speak these Scriptures over yourself. Doing this will build your faith for your healthy pregnancies and children.

All Scripture references are from the Amplified translation of the Bible, unless otherwise noted.

Genesis 1:27-28
So God created man in His own image, in the image and likeness of God He created him; male and female He created them.

And God blessed them and said to them, Be fruitful, multiply, and fill the earth, and subdue it [using all its vast resources in the service of God and man]; and have dominion over the fish of the sea, the birds of the air, and over every living creature that moves upon the earth.

Genesis 9:7
And you, be fruitful and multiply; bring forth abundantly on the earth and multiply on it.

Genesis 15:2-6

And Abram said, Lord God, what can You give me, since I am going on [from this world] childless and he who shall be the owner and heir of my house is this [steward] Eliezer of Damascus?

And Abram continued, Look, You have given me no child; and [a servant] born in my house is my heir.

And behold, the word of the Lord came to him, saying, This man shall not be your heir, but he who shall come from your own body shall be your heir.

And He brought him outside [his tent into the starlight] and said, Look now toward the heavens and count the stars—if you are able to number them. Then He said to him, So shall your descendants be.

And he [Abram] believed in (trusted in, relied on, remained steadfast to) the Lord, and He counted it to him as righteousness (right standing with God).

Genesis 17:15-17

And God said to Abraham, As for Sarai your wife, you shall not call her name Sarai; but Sarah [Princess] her name shall be.

And I will bless her and give you a son also by her. Yes, I will bless her, and she shall be a mother of nations; kings of peoples shall come from her.

Then Abraham fell on his face and laughed and said in his heart, Shall a child be born to a man who is a hundred years old? And shall Sarah, who is ninety years old, bear a son?

Genesis 21:7

And she said, Who would have said to Abraham that Sarah would nurse children at the breast? For I have borne him a son in his old age!

Genesis 25:21

And Isaac prayed much to the Lord for his wife because she was unable to bear children; and the Lord granted his prayer, and Rebekah his wife became pregnant.

Genesis 30:22-24

Then God remembered Rachel and answered her pleading and made it possible for her to have children.

And [now for the first time] she became pregnant and bore a son; and she said, God has taken away my reproach, disgrace, and humiliation.

And she called his name Joseph [may he add] and said, May the Lord add to me another son.

Exodus 13:2

Sanctify (consecrate, set apart) to Me all the firstborn [males]; whatever is first to open the womb among the Israelites, both of man and of beast, is Mine.

Exodus 23:26

None shall lose her young by miscarriage or be barren in your land; I will fulfill the number of your days.

Deuteronomy 7:13-14

And He will love you, bless you, and multiply you; He will also bless the fruit of your body and the fruit of your land, your grain, your new wine, and your oil, the increase of your cattle and the young of your flock in the land which He swore to your fathers to give you.

You shall be blessed above all peoples; there shall not be male or female barren among you, or among your cattle.

Judges 13:2-3, 5 & 24

And there was a certain man of Zorah, of the tribe of the Danites, whose name was Manoah; and his wife was barren and had no children.

And the Angel of the Lord appeared to the woman and said to her, Behold, you are barren and have no children, but you shall become pregnant and bear a son.

For behold, you shall become pregnant and bear a son. No razor shall come upon his head, for the child shall be a Nazirite to God from birth, and he shall begin to deliver Israel out of the hands of the Philistines.

And the woman [in due time] bore a son and called his name Samson; and the child grew and the Lord blessed him.

1 Samuel 1:26-28

Hannah said, Oh, my lord! As your soul lives, my lord, I am the woman who stood by you here praying to the Lord.

For this child I prayed, and the Lord has granted my petition made to Him.

Therefore I have given him to the Lord; as long as he lives he is given to the Lord. And they worshiped the Lord there.

1 Samuel 2:20-21

And Eli would bless Elkanah and his wife and say, May the Lord give you children by this woman for the gift she asked for and gave to the Lord. Then they would go to their own home.

And the Lord visited Hannah, so that she bore three sons and two daughters. And the child Samuel grew before the Lord.

2 Kings 2:19-21

And the men of the city said to Elisha, Behold, inhabiting of this city is pleasant, as my lord sees, but the water is bad and the locality causes miscarriage and barrenness [in all animals].

He said, Bring me a new bowl and put salt [the symbol of God's purifying power] in it. And they brought it to him.

Then Elisha went to the spring of the waters and cast the salt in it and said, Thus says the Lord: I [not the salt] have healed these waters; there shall not be any more death, miscarriage or barrenness [and bereavement] because of it.

2 Kings 4:13-17

And he said to Gehazi, Say now to her, You have been most painstakingly and reverently concerned for us; what is to be done for you? Would you like to be spoken for to the king or to the commander of the army? She answered, I dwell among my own people [they are sufficient].

Later Elisha said, What then is to be done for her? Gehazi answered, She has no child and her husband is old.

He said, Call her. [Gehazi] called her, and she stood in the doorway.

Elisha said, At this season when the time comes round, you shall embrace a son. She said, No, my lord, you man of God, do not lie to your handmaid.

But the woman conceived and bore a son at that season the following year, as Elisha had said to her.

Psalm 37:4

Delight yourself also in the Lord, and He will give you the desires and secret petitions of your heart.

Psalm 128:1-3

Blessed (happy, fortunate, to be envied) is everyone who fears, reveres, and worships the Lord, who walks in His ways and lives according to His commandments.

For you shall eat [the fruit] of the labor of your hands; happy (blessed, fortunate, enviable) shall you be, and it shall be well with you.

Your wife shall be like a fruitful vine in the innermost parts of your house; your children shall be like olive plants round about your table.

Psalm 138:8
The Lord will accomplish that which concerns me; Your (unwavering) loving kindness, O Lord, endures forever–Do not abandon the works of Your own hands.

Psalm 139:13-16
For You did form my inward parts; You did knit me together in my mother's womb.

I will confess and praise You for You are fearful and wonderful and for the awful wonder of my birth! Wonderful are Your works, and that my inner self knows right well.

My frame was not hidden from You when I was being formed in secret [and] intricately and curiously wrought [as if embroidered with various colors] in the depths of the earth [a region of darkness and mystery].

Your eyes saw my unformed substance, and in Your book all the days [of my life] were written before ever they took shape, when as yet there was none of them.

Ecclesiastes 11:5

As you know not what is the way of the wind, or how the spirit comes to the bones in the womb of a pregnant woman, even so you know not the work of God, Who does all.

Isaiah 44:24

24Thus says the Lord, your Redeemer, and He Who formed you from the womb: I am the Lord, Who made all things, Who alone stretched out the heavens, Who spread out the earth by Myself [who was with Me]?

Isaiah 49:1

Listen to me, O isles and coast lands, and hearken, you peoples from afar. The Lord has called me from the womb; from the body of my mother He has named my name.

Isaiah 65:23

They shall not labor in vain or bring forth [children] for sudden terror or calamity; for they shall be the descendants of the blessed of the Lord, and their offspring with them.

Luke 1:6-7, 13-14

And they both were righteous in the sight of God, walking blamelessly in all the commandments and requirements of the Lord.

But they had no child, for Elizabeth was barren; and both were far advanced in years.

But the angel said to him, Do not be afraid, Zachariah, because your petition was heard, and your wife Elizabeth will bear you a son, and you must call his name John [God is favorable].

And you shall have joy and exultant delight, and many will rejoice over his birth,

Luke 1:36-37

And listen! Your relative Elizabeth in her old age has also conceived a son, and this is now the sixth month with her who was called barren.

For with God nothing is ever impossible and no word from God shall be without power or impossible of fulfillment.

Luke 2:23

As it is written in the Law of the Lord, Every [firstborn] male that opens the womb shall be set apart and dedicated and called holy to the Lord

Mark 11:23-24

Truly I tell you, whoever says to this mountain, Be lifted up and thrown into the sea! and does not doubt at all in his heart but believes that what he says will take place, it will be done for him.

For this reason I am telling you, whatever you ask for in prayer, believe (trust and be confident) that it is granted to you, and you will [get it].

Romans 4:18-20

[For Abraham, human reason for] hope being gone, hoped in faith that he should become the father of many nations, as he had been promised, So [numberless] shall your descendants be.

He did not weaken in faith when he considered the [utter] impotence of his own body, which was as good as dead because he was about a hundred years old, or [when he considered] the barrenness of Sarah's [deadened] womb.

No unbelief or distrust made him waver (doubtingly question) concerning the promise of God, but he grew strong and was empowered by faith as he gave praise and glory to God,

Hebrews 11:11

Because of faith also Sarah herself received physical power to conceive a child, even when she was long past the age for it, because she considered [God] Who had given her the promise to be reliable and trustworthy and true to His word.

Hebrews 4:12

For the Word that God speaks is alive and full of power [making it active, operative, energizing, and effective]; it is sharper than any two-edged sword, penetrating to the dividing line of the breath of life (soul) and [the immortal] spirit, and of joints and marrow [of the deepest parts of our nature], exposing and sifting and analyzing and judging the very thoughts and purposes of the heart.

www.ingramcontent.com/pod-product-compliance
Lightning Source LLC
LaVergne TN
LVHW010504160826
845677LV00012B/2642

* 9 7 9 8 3 7 4 5 5 7 2 4 4 *